Steroids and Other Appearance and Performance Enhancing Drugs (APEDs)

Table of Contents

Introduction

Appearance and performance enhancing drugs (APEDs) are most often used by males to improve appearance by building muscle mass or to enhance athletic performance. Although they may directly and indirectly have effects on a user's mood, they do not produce a euphoric high, which makes APEDs distinct from other drugs such as cocaine, heroin, and marijuana. However, users may develop a substance use disorder, defined as continued use despite adverse consequences.

Anabolic-androgenic steroids, the best-studied class of APEDs (and the main subject of this report) can boost a user's confidence and strength, leading users to overlook the severe, long-lasting, and in some cases, irreversible damage they can cause. They can lead to early heart attacks, strokes, liver tumors, kidney failure, and psychiatric problems. In addition, stopping use can cause depression, often leading to resumption of use.

Because steroids are often injected, users who share needles or use nonsterile injecting techniques are also at risk for contracting dangerous infections such as viral hepatitis and HIV.

Steroids are popularly associated with doping by elite athletes, but since the 1980s, their use by male non-athlete weightlifters has exceeded their use by competitive athletes.[1] Their use is closely associated with disordered male body image—most specifically, muscle dysmorphia.

What are the different types of APEDs?

Anabolic-androgenic steroids, often shortened to "anabolic steroids," "steroids," or "androgens,"[2,3] are the most widely misused APED. These are synthetic substances similar to the male sex hormone testosterone. They promote the growth of skeletal muscle (anabolic effects) and the development of male sexual characteristics (androgenic effects) in both males and females.[2]

These compounds are sometimes used medically to treat delayed puberty and muscle loss due to disease[4] and to treat low levels of testosterone in men with an associated medical condition.[5] Anabolic androgenic steroids can also improve feelings of well-being and increase bone strength, but are not approved for these purposes. However, testosterone-supplementation therapy is an increasingly common treatment for mood and sexual performance problems associated with male aging, and it is controversially being prescribed even for younger men.[6]

Note that in the context of this report, anabolic steroids refer only to the non-prescribed use (misuse) of testosterone and testosterone-like substances by athletes and non-athlete bodybuilders. This research report will not cover image enhancers, such as dermal fillers, Botox, or the skin tanner, melanotan.[7]

Non-steroidal anabolics, include insulin, insulin-like growth hormone (IGF), and human growth hormone (HGH)—substances that are produced by the human body and are prescribed for legitimate medical uses but also sometimes misused for performance enhancement.

Ergo/thermogenics are compounds used to decrease body fat or to promote leanness versus muscle mass in endurance athletes.[8] The three main categories of ergo/thermogenics are:

- **Xanthines**: compounds that increase attention and wakefulness and suppress appetite. Examples are caffeine, the asthma drug theophylline, and theobromine—a substance found in chocolate, coffee, and tea.[9]

- **Sympathomimetics**: drugs that are similar in structure and action to epinephrine and norepinephrine—natural chemicals in the body that increase heart rate, constrict blood vessels, and raise blood pressure. An example is ephedrine, which is derived from the ephedra plant. Ephedrine/ephedra used to be included in dietary supplements that promoted weight loss, increased energy, and enhanced athletic performance.[10] In 2004, the FDA banned the U.S. sale of dietary supplements containing ephedrine/ephedra due to various possible health risks including cardiovascular and nervous system effects.[11]

- **Thyroid hormones**: substances that regulate metabolism by altering the function of the thyroid.[12] Cytomel is an example.

Nutritional/dietary supplements are substances purchased legally from nutritional stores or via the internet that are often taken in combination with other APEDS. Creatine, which boosts exercise capacity, is one common example.

In the United States, dietary supplements containing steroid precursors such as tetrahydrogestrinone (THG) and androstenedione (street name "Andro") previously could be purchased legally without a prescription. Athletes took steroid precursors in an effort to boost testosterone levels. Less is known about the side effects of steroid precursors, but if large quantities of these compounds substantially increase testosterone levels in the body, then they also are likely to produce the same side effects as anabolic steroids themselves.[13] The purchase of these supplements, with the notable exception of dehydroepiandrosterone (DHEA), became illegal after the passage of the Anabolic Steroid Control Act of 2004, which amended the Controlled Substances Act.[14]

What is the history of anabolic steroid use?

Testosterone was first synthesized in Germany in 1935[15] and was used medically to treat depression.[16] Professional athletes began misusing anabolic steroids during the 1954 Olympics, when Russian weightlifters were given testosterone.[17] In the 1980s, anabolic steroid use began to extend into the general population, and young men began using these substances, sometimes to enhance athletic performance but in most cases to improve personal appearance.[18]

Most anabolic steroid users are male non-athletes aiming to improve their appearance by building muscle, and use of steroids is strongly tied to a male body image disorder called muscle dysmorphia (see "Who uses anabolic steroids?").[19] Just as female body image disorders have been linked to unrealistic portrayals of the female form in fashion magazines and popular culture, muscle dysmorphia in males is linked to exaggerated physiques in action movies and other media over the past three decades.[19]

Congress passed the Anabolic Steroid Act of 1990 to respond to the increasing levels of illicit traffic in steroids. This Act identified anabolic steroids as a separate drug class and categorized over two dozen drugs as controlled substances. The Act also gave a four-part definition of this drug class, which allowed for flexibility in controlling new anabolic steroids as they were synthesized. In 2004, Congress enacted the Anabolic Steroid Control Act of 2004, which banned over-the-counter steroid precursors; increased penalties for making, selling, or possessing illegal steroid precursors; and provided funds for preventative educational efforts.[20]

Other countries, such as Mexico and some European nations, where steroids are available without prescription, are the main sources of illegal steroids smuggled into the United States. Less common illicit sources include diversion from legitimate sources (e.g., thefts or inappropriate prescribing) or production within clandestine laboratories.[21]

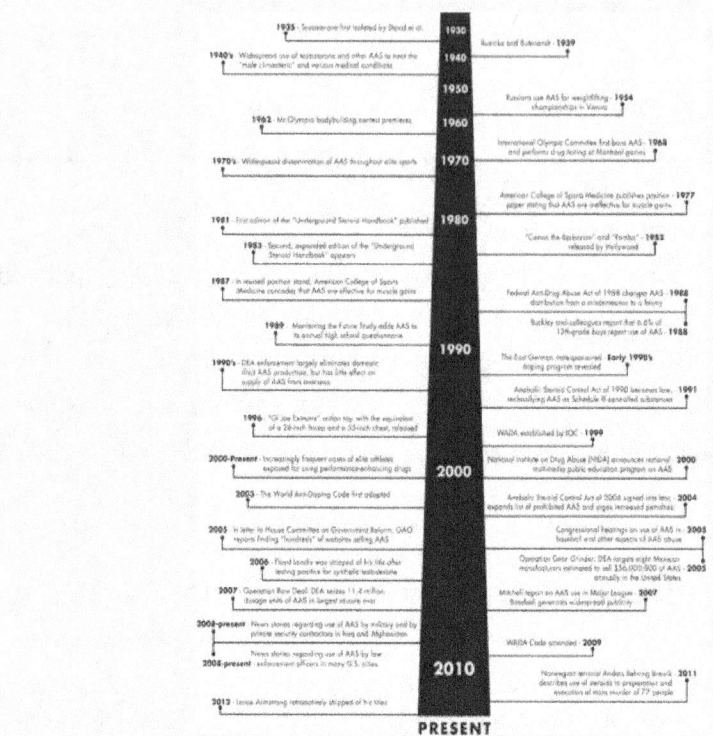

A historical timeline of anabolic steroids.

Source: Pope, Wood, Rogol, Nyberg, Bowers, Bhasin. *Endocrine Reviews*. 2014.

Who uses anabolic steroids?

The vast majority of people who misuse steroids are male non-athlete weightlifters in their 20s or 30s.[1,22] Contrary to popular belief, only about 22 percent of anabolic steroid users started as teenagers.[23] Anabolic steroid use is less common among females, since fewer women desire extreme muscularity and the masculinizing effects of steroids.[22]

Males who are more likely to use steroids tend to have poor self-esteem, higher rates of depression, more suicide attempts, poor knowledge and attitudes about health, greater participation in sports emphasizing weight and shape, greater parental concern about weight, and higher rates of eating disorders and substance use.[24] Steroid misuse is associated with muscle dysmorphia, a behavioral disorder in which men think that they look small and weak, even if they are large and muscular (see "Why are anabolic steroids misused?").[25]

Some people who misuse steroids have experienced physical or sexual abuse. In a study of 506 male users and 771 male nonusers of anabolic steroids, users were significantly more likely than nonusers to report being sexually abused in the past.[26] Similarly, female weightlifters who had been raped were found to be twice as likely to report use of anabolic steroids or another purported muscle-building drug, compared with those who had not been raped. Moreover, almost all females who had been raped reported that they markedly increased their bodybuilding activities after the attack. They believed that being bigger and stronger would discourage further attacks because men would find them either intimidating or unattractive.[27]

It is difficult to estimate the true prevalence of steroid misuse in the United States because many surveys that ask about illicit drug use do not include questions about steroids. However, the annual Monitoring the Future study, a NIDA-funded survey of drug use and attitudes in middle and high school students across the United States, shows that past-year use of steroids has generally declined among 8th and 10th graders, after peaking in 2000. Past-year steroid use among 12th graders increased from 2011 to 2015, although use significantly declined from 2015 to 2016. The 2017 rate of use among 12th graders holds relatively steady.

Past Year Anabolic Steroid Use Among Middle and High School Students, 2007-2017

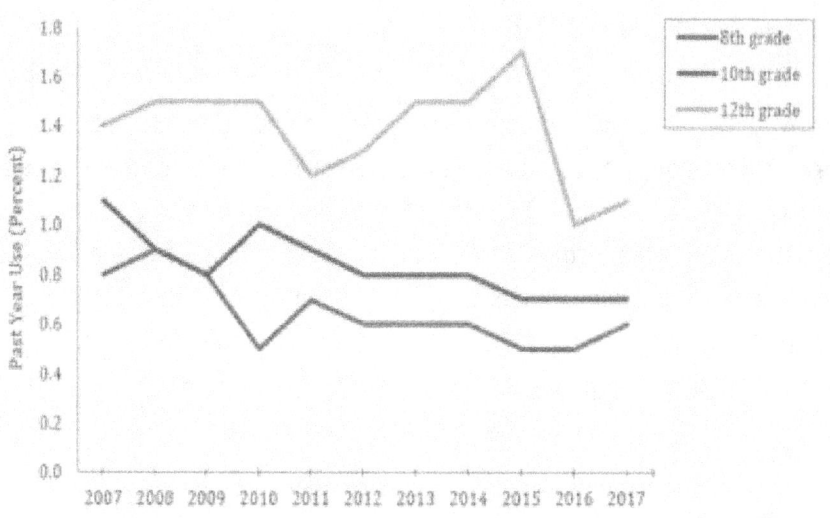

Data are from the 2017 Monitoring the Future survey, funded by the National Institute on Drug Abuse and conducted annually by the University of Michigan's Institute for Social Research.

Why are anabolic steroids misused?

Anabolic steroids increase lean muscle mass when used in conjunction with weight training. The aim, for non-athlete weightlifters, is typically improvement of appearance. As mentioned in "Who uses anabolic steroids?" steroid use is often associated with a form of male body dysmorphic disorder called muscle dysmorphia, a preoccupation with the perceived inadequate size of their muscles.[19]

As a result, some users report taking anabolic steroids to increase confidence and because they feel that they are at a point where they can no longer get bigger through weight training alone. Most users report that anabolic steroids help them achieve their ideal body.[28]

Increasing muscle mass may also promote strength, which can improve performance in certain types of sports. More benefit is seen for strength-dependent sports (weightlifting, shot-put throwing, football) than for sports that require speed, agility, flexibility, and/or endurance.[29]

Anabolic steroid users also report that their muscles recover faster from intense strain and muscle injury.[30] Research in animals has not conclusively supported this belief, with some showing that anabolic steroids can enhance recovery from certain types of muscle damage,[31,32] but others finding no benefit in taking anabolic steroids to enhance muscle recovery.[33]

Anabolic steroid users report using an average of about 11 APEDs per year. They are also more likely than non-steroid users to take supplements such as protein powders and creatine; estrogen blockers; ergo/thermogenics, such as caffeine or ephedrine; medications for erectile dysfunction; and other hormones such as insulin, thyroid hormones, and human growth hormone.[26]

How are anabolic steroids used?

Some anabolic steroids are taken orally, others are injected intramuscularly,[29] and still others are provided in gels or creams that are applied to the skin.[35] Many users start with the oral form and then progress to injectable forms,[36] since the latter causes less liver damage. However, oral steroids clear more rapidly from the body, often making this the preferred route for users concerned with drug testing.[29] Doses taken by people misusing these substances can be 10 to 100 times higher than the doses used to treat medical conditions.[36]

Commonly Misused Steroids

Oral Steroids

- Anadrol (oxymetholone)

- Anavar (oxandrolone)

- Dianabol (methandienone)

- Winstrol (stanozolol)

- Restandol (testosterone undecanoate)

Injectable Steroids

- Deca-Durabolin (nandrolone decanoate)

- Durabolin (nandrolone phenpropionate)

- Depo-Testosterone (testosterone cypionate)

- Agovirin (testosterone propionate)

- Retandrol (testosterone phenylpropionate)

- Equipoise (boldenone undecylenate)[29,34]

Cycling, stacking, pyramiding, and plateauing

Steroids are often used in patterns called "cycling." This involves taking multiple doses of steroids over a specific period of time, stopping for a period, and starting again. People who misuse steroids also typically "stack" the drugs, meaning that they take two or more different anabolic steroids, mix oral and/or injectable types, and sometimes even take compounds that are designed for veterinary use.[37,38] The belief is that different steroids interact to produce an effect on muscle size that is greater than the effects of each drug individually,[36] a theory that has not been tested scientifically.

Another common mode of steroid misuse is referred to as "pyramiding," which typically involves taking them in a cycle of six to 12 weeks, tapering gradually rather than starting and finishing a cycle abruptly. At the beginning of a cycle, the person starts with low doses of the drugs being stacked and then slowly increases the doses. In the second half of the cycle, the doses are slowly decreased to zero. This is sometimes followed by a second cycle in which the person continues to train but without drugs. Steroid users believe that pyramiding allows the body time to adjust to the high doses, and the drug-free cycle allows the body's hormonal system time to recuperate.[2]

A technique called "plateauing" may also be used, whereby steroids are staggered, overlapped, or substituted with another type of steroid to avoid developing tolerance.[36] As with stacking, the effects of pyramiding, cycling, and plateauing have not been substantiated scientifically.

What are the side effects of anabolic steroid misuse?

A variety of side effects can occur when anabolic steroids are misused, ranging from mild effects to ones that are harmful or even life-threatening. Most are reversible if the user stops taking the drugs. However, others may be permanent or semi-permanent.

Most data on the long-term effects of anabolic steroids in humans come from case reports rather than formal epidemiological studies. Serious and life-threatening adverse effects may be underreported, especially since they may occur many years later. One review found 19 deaths in published case reports related to anabolic steroid use between 1990 and 2012; however, many steroid users also used other drugs, making it difficult to show that the anabolic steroid use caused these deaths.[39] One animal study found that exposing male mice for one fifth of their lifespan to steroid doses comparable to those taken by human athletes caused a high frequency of early deaths.[40]

Possible Health Consequences of Anabolic Steroid Misuse

Cardiovascular system

- high blood pressure
- blood clots
- heart attacks
- stroke
- artery damage

Hormonal system

Men

- decreased sperm production
- enlarged breasts
- shrinking of the testicles
- male-pattern baldness
- testicular cancer

Women

- voice deepening
- decreased breast size
- coarse skin
- excessive body hair growth
- male-pattern baldness

Infection

- HIV/AIDS
- hepatitis

Liver

- peliosis hepatis
- tumors

Musculoskeletal system

- short stature (if taken by adolescents)
- tendon injury

Psychiatric effects

- aggression
- mania
- delusions

Skin

- severe acne and cysts
- oily scalp and skin
- abscess at injection site
- jaundice

Cardiovascular System

Steroid use has been associated with high blood pressure;[41] decreased function of the heart's ventricles;[23,41,42] and cardiovascular diseases such as heart attacks,[43] artery damage,[44] and strokes,[45,46] even in athletes younger than 30. Steroids contribute to the development of cardiovascular disease partly by increasing the level of low-density lipoprotein (LDL)[47] and decreasing the level of high-density lipoprotein (HDL).[47,48] High LDL and low HDL levels increase the risk of atherosclerosis, a condition in which fatty substances are deposited inside arteries and disrupt blood flow. If blood is prevented from reaching the heart or brain, the result can be a heart attack or stroke, respectively. Steroids also increase the risk that blood clots will form in blood vessels, potentially disrupting blood flow and damaging the heart muscle, so that it does not pump blood effectively.[49]

Hormonal System

Steroid use disrupts the normal production of hormones in the body. Changes that can be reversed include decreased sperm production,[56-59] decreased function of the testes (hypogonadism) that leads to low testosterone levels,[60] and shrinking of the testicles (testicular atrophy).[56,61] Irreversible changes include male-pattern baldness and breast development (gynecomastia) in men.[59,62] Anabolic steroids may also act upon the hormone system to increase the risk of testicular cancer, especially when steroids are used in combination with insulin-like growth factor.[63]

In females, anabolic steroids cause masculinization. Specifically, breast size and body fat decrease, the skin becomes coarse, and the voice deepens.[64] Women may experience excessive growth of body hair but lose scalp hair.[65] With continued administration of steroids, some of these effects become irreversible. It is commonly believed that anabolic steroids will produce irreversible enlargement of the clitoris in females, although there are no studies on this.[66]

Infections

Many people who inject anabolic steroids may use nonsterile injection techniques or share contaminated needles with other users. This puts these steroid users at risk for acquiring life threatening viral infections, such as HIV and hepatitis B and C.[76] In addition, animal models indicate that anabolic steroids suppress the immune system,[77] which could worsen infections.

Liver

Steroid misuse has been associated with liver damage,[50,51] tumors,[46,52,53] and a rare condition called peliosis hepatis, in which blood-filled cysts form in the liver.[54] The cysts can rupture, causing internal bleeding and even death in rare cases.[55]

Musculoskeletal System

Rising levels of testosterone and other sex hormones normally trigger the growth spurt that occurs during puberty and adolescence. These rising levels of testosterone also provide the signals to stop growth.[67] When a child or adolescent takes anabolic steroids, the resulting artificially high sex hormone levels can prematurely signal the bones to stop growing.[68]

Evidence suggests that weightlifters who misuse anabolic steroids have stiffer tendons, which could lead to an increased risk for tendon injury.[69]

Skin

Steroid misuse can cause acne,[70–72] hair loss on the head, cysts, and oily hair and skin.[65] Users who inject steroids may also develop pain and abscess formation at injection sites.[73]

Anabolic steroids can also produce jaundice, or yellowing of the skin or eyes, as a result of damage to the liver.[74,75]

How does anabolic steroid misuse affect behavior?

Aggression

Case reports and small studies indicate that anabolic steroids increase irritability and aggression,[75] although findings may be confounded by personality traits that are overrepresented in steroid users (i.e., antisocial, borderline, and histrionic personality disorder)[78] and use of other drugs.[79] People who misuse anabolic steroids report more anger than nonusers,[80] as well as more fights, verbal aggression, and violence toward their significant others,[81] sometimes called "roid rage." One study suggests that the mood and behavioral effects seen during anabolic-androgenic steroid misuse may result from secondary hormonal changes.[82]

Scientists have attempted to test the association between anabolic steroids and aggression by administering high steroid doses or placebo for days or weeks to human volunteers and then assessing behavioral symptoms. In one such study, researchers found that testosterone over a six week period was associated with increased aggression, as assessed by a questionnaire and computer-based model of aggressive behavior.[83] In addition, high steroid doses produced greater feelings of irritability and aggression than placebo,[84] although the effects appear to be highly variable across individuals,[19] and other studies have not shown that effect.[85] One possible explanation, according to the researchers, is that some but not all anabolic steroids increase irritability and aggression.

Psychiatric Disorders

Anabolic steroid users are more likely than nonusers to report anxiety.[34,86] Moderate to high doses of anabolic steroids are also associated with major mood disorders such as mania, hypomania,[87] and major depression.[86,87] In one study, manic symptoms were not uniform across individuals, with most showing little psychological change, whereas a few demonstrated prominent effects.[19]

Other Drug Use

Anabolic steroid users are more likely to use drugs such as marijuana, prescription opioids, cocaine,[88] or heroin.[86] In a study of men admitted to treatment for opioid use disorders, 25 percent reported prior use of anabolic steroids. Some described first learning about opioids from friends at the gym, and that they first purchased opioids from the same person who had sold them the anabolic steroids.[89] In a study of anabolic steroid users dependent upon the injectable opioid analgesic nalbuphine, most reported that they began using nalbuphine to treat pain from weightlifting injuries. They also described widespread use of nalbuphine in their gyms.[90]

Research also indicates that some users might turn to other drugs to alleviate some of the negative effects of anabolic steroids. For example, a study of 227 men admitted in 1999 to a private treatment center for addiction to heroin or other opioids found that 9.3 percent had previously misused anabolic steroids. Of these, most reported using opioids to counteract insomnia, irritability, depression, and withdrawal from anabolic steroids.[91]

What are the risks of anabolic steroid use in teens?

Unlike most illicit drug use, misuse of anabolic steroids most commonly begins in young adulthood rather than adolescence. But steroid use in teens is of concern, especially since the hormonal systems they interact with play a critical role in brain development during these years.[92–96] In adolescent rodents, exposure to anabolic steroids increased neuronal spine densities in the hippocampus and amygdala—brain regions involved in learning and emotions (e.g., aggression), respectively. Four weeks after withdrawal, these increases in neuronal spine densities returned to normal in the amygdala, but not in the hippocampus. This suggests that pubertal steroid exposure could produce long-lasting structural changes in certain brain regions.[97]

Teens who use anabolic steroids may also be at increased risk for some cognitive side effects compared with adults. For example, males who begin using anabolic steroids during the teen years show increased impulsivity and decreased attention, compared to men who began using steroids in their adult years.[98] In adolescent rats, anabolic steroid exposure is associated with electrolytic imbalances, hyperactivity, anxiety, and increased sympathetic autonomic modulation (e.g., fight or flight response) during adulthood, even when steroid use was discontinued during adolescence.[99] In addition, adolescent male hamsters given anabolic steroids show increased aggression, even after steroid use is discontinued. These aggressive effects are paralleled by changes in levels of serotonin[100,101] and androgen receptors in the rodent brain.[102]

How do anabolic steroids work in the brain?

Anabolic steroids act at androgen receptors to influence cellular functioning and gene expression. In addition to regulating pathways involved in the development of male characteristics,[103] activation of androgen receptors also produces rapid increases in calcium levels within skeletal muscle, heart, and brain cells.[104] Calcium plays important roles in neuronal signaling.

Research with human cells demonstrates that anabolic steroids also interact with certain types of $GABA_A$ receptors, which could mediate the increased anxiety reported by steroid users.[105,106] In addition, animal studies show that anabolic steroids increase serotonin levels in brain regions involved in mood[107] and dopamine levels in reward-related brain regions.[107,108] Chronic use of anabolic steroids has also been shown to cause dysfunction of these reward pathways in animals. Specifically, rats given twice daily nandrolone injections for four weeks showed loss of sweet preference (a sign of reward dysfunction) that was accompanied by reductions of dopamine, serotonin, and noradrenaline in the nucleus accumbens, a reward-related brain region.[109]

Are anabolic steroids addictive?

An undetermined percentage of steroid users may develop a steroid use disorder. Substance use disorders are defined by continued use despite adverse consequences; for steroid users, these may include physical or psychological problems such as breast growth (in men), sexual dysfunction, high blood pressure, excessive fats in the blood, heart disease, mood swings, severe irritability, or aggressiveness. Anabolic steroid users also may give up other important activities for fear that they will miss workouts, violate their dietary restrictions, or be prevented from using steroids. Steroid users also typically spend large amounts of time and money obtaining the drugs, and they may try to reduce or stop anabolic steroid use without success—possibly due to depression, anxiety about losing muscle mass, or and other unpleasant effects of withdrawal.[110]

Withdrawal from steroids occurs when an individual develops dependence. A review of the research suggests that about 32 percent of people who misuse anabolic steroids become dependent.[23] Symptoms of dependence can include tolerance, which is needing to take more steroids to achieve the same effects. Another indicator of dependence is withdrawal once anabolic steroid use stops.[110] Withdrawal symptoms can include fatigue, restlessness, loss of appetite, insomnia, reduced sex drive, and steroid cravings.[111] The most dangerous of the withdrawal symptoms is depression, because it sometimes leads to suicide attempts.[112]

How are anabolic steroids tested in athletes?

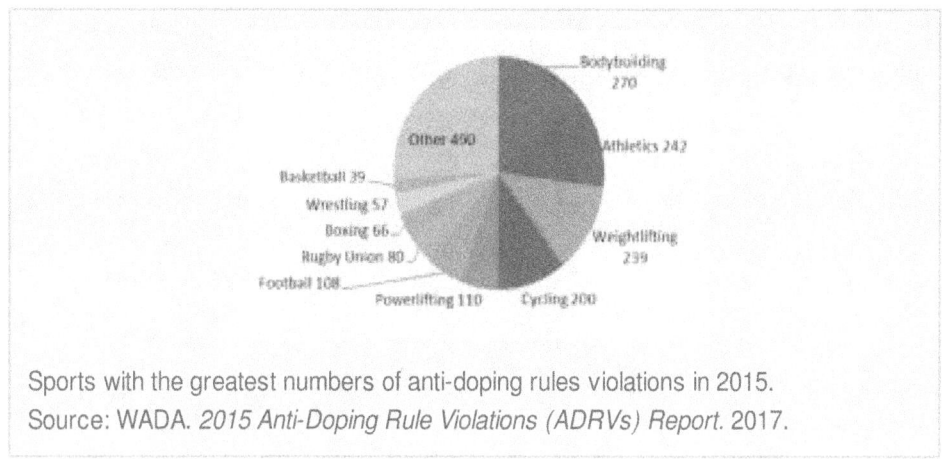

Sports with the greatest numbers of anti-doping rules violations in 2015.
Source: WADA. *2015 Anti-Doping Rule Violations (ADRVs) Report.* 2017.

Although non-athlete weightlifters account for the bulk of anabolic steroid misuse, occasional steroid use by professional and Olympic athletes to improve performance or cheat in competition ("doping") has done the most to raise awareness of steroid misuse. The World Anti-Doping Agency (WADA) was founded in 1999 to consistently apply anti-doping policies across sports organizations and governments around the world. Non-compliant organizations can face sanctions such as event cancellation, loss of WADA funding, or ineligibility to host events.[114]

Refinements in drug testing have improved the ability to detect anti-doping violations, resulting in increased numbers of reported violations over recent years. For example, the discovery of long-term steroid metabolites has lengthened the drug detection window, making it more difficult for athletes to pass drug tests by simply discontinuing steroid use just prior to an event. In addition, more sensitive technologies have allowed detection of lower metabolite thresholds.[115]

Although testing procedures are now in place to deter steroid use among professional and Olympic athletes, new designer drugs constantly become available that can escape detection and put athletes willing to cheat one step ahead of testing efforts.[116–118] To detect early use of designer steroids and provide more accurate baseline standards for each athlete, testing laboratories store data from each drug testing sample. These samples are then used as reference points for future testing, thereby eliminating the possibility that a person tests positive simply because he or she has naturally elevated levels of testosterone when compared to the general population.[119] Long-term use of designer steroids suppresses levels endogenous steroids in urine samples, which could be the first indication that an athlete is taking a designer steroid.[117]

Drug Testing and Nutritional Supplements

Athletes taking over-the-counter nutritional supplements may believe that such products are safe. However, nutritional supplements are not subjected to the same pre-approval requirements and quality tests as FDA-approved medications.[120] For example, some supplements advertised to promote weight loss have been found to contain banned stimulants such as ephedrine[121] or clenbuterol.[122] Other research shows that supplements sometimes contain prohormones or anabolic steroids.[123] In a study looking at 634 nutritional supplements from 13 different countries, 15 percent included some type of prohormone not listed on the label.[115] Another study showed that some non-labeled prohibited substances could be detected by drug tests up to 144 hours later.[124]

Nutritional supplements sometimes contain banned substances that are not indicated in their labels.[115,124] The FDA notes that consumers should be wary if a product meets any of these criteria:

- products claiming to be alternatives to FDA-approved drugs or to have effects similar to prescription drugs

- products claiming to be a legal alternative to anabolic steroids

- products that are marketed primarily in a foreign language or those that are marketed through mass e-mails

- sexual enhancement products promising rapid effects such as working in minutes to hours, or long-lasting effects such as 24 hours to 72 hours

- products that provide warnings about testing positive in performance enhancement drug tests[125]

According to WADA's codes, athletes are responsible for any prohibited substance found in their samples, regardless of whether ingestion was intentional or unintentional. However, sanctions may be reduced or avoided if the athlete can demonstrate that the substance was ingested through no significant fault or negligence on his/her part, or in some circumstances where the athlete did not intend to enhance performance.[126]

What can be done to prevent steroid misuse?

Research suggests that high school athletes are less likely to use steroids if their peers and parents disapprove, indicating that peers and parents can be strong partners in prevention efforts.[127]

However, research shows that simply teaching students about steroids' adverse effects does not convince adolescents that they will be adversely affected, nor does such instruction discourage young people from taking steroids in the future. Presenting both the risks and benefits of anabolic steroid use is more effective in convincing adolescents about steroids' negative effects, apparently because the students find a balanced approach more credible.[128]

Research also indicates that some adolescents misuse steroids as part of a pattern of high-risk behaviors such as drinking and driving, carrying a gun, driving a motorcycle without a helmet, and using other illicit drugs. This suggests that a prevention program should focus on comprehensive high-risk behavior screening and counseling among teens who use anabolic steroids.[129]

NIDA-Funded Prevention Research Helps Reduce Steroid Misuse

A more sophisticated approach has shown promise for preventing steroid misuse among players on high school sports teams. The Adolescents Training and Learning to Avoid Steroids (ATLAS) program is showing high school football players that they do not need steroids to build powerful muscles and improve athletic performance. By educating student athletes about the harmful effects of anabolic steroids and providing nutrition and weight-training alternatives to steroid use, the ATLAS program has increased football players' healthy behaviors and reduced their intentions to misuse steroids. In the program, coaches and team leaders teach the harmful effects of anabolic steroids and other illicit drugs on immediate sports performance and discuss how to refuse offers of drugs.[130]

Studies show that one year after completion of the program, compared with a control group, ATLAS-trained football student athletes in 15 high schools had:

- less use of anabolic steroids and less intention to misuse them in the future

- less misuse of alcohol, amphetamines, and narcotics

- less misuse of "athletic enhancing" supplements

- less likelihood of engaging in hazardous behaviors such as drinking and driving

- better knowledge about anabolic steroid, alcohol, and marijuana effects; better knowledge of alternatives to steroid misuse; greater confidence in athletic abilities; and improved nutritional behaviors[130]

The Athletes Targeting Healthy Exercise and Nutrition Alternatives (ATHENA) program was patterned after the ATLAS program, but designed for adolescent girls on sports teams. Early testing of girls enrolled in the ATHENA program showed significant decreases compared to controls in risky behaviors such as riding with an intoxicated driver or engaging in sexual activity with new partners. ATHENA participants were also less likely to use diet pills, amphetamines, anabolic steroids, and muscle-building supplements during the sports season. Although the program had no immediate effect on tobacco, alcohol, or marijuana use,[131] ATHENA-trained athletes reported less lifetime use of these substances when surveyed one to three years following high school graduation. Diet pill and steroid use declined by this one to three year follow-up for both ATHENA-trained and control-group athletes, so that these groups no longer differed in their use of these substances.[132]

What treatments are effective for anabolic steroid misuse?

People who use steroids often do not seek treatment for their use, with one study reporting that 56 percent of users had never told their physician about their use.[133] This could be because users feel their physician lacks knowledge about anabolic steroids.[133] In addition, many internet sites devoted to anabolic steroids and other APEDs challenge the professionalism of health care providers and offer their own medically questionable advice on the use of APEDs.[134] This makes it important for health care providers to be educated on the signs and symptoms of steroid use in their patients.[111]

Current views recommend that treatment for steroid use address the underlying causes of the steroid use. This can include:

- psychological therapies (and possibly medications) for muscle dysmorphia

- endocrine therapies to restore function in those suffering from hypogonadism and to alleviate symptoms of depression

- antidepressants for those whose depression does not respond to endocrine therapies

- pharmacological and psychosocial treatments for patients who are also dependent on opioids, which appear to also be effective in alleviating signs of anabolic steroid dependence[135]

Where can I get further information about steroids?

To learn more about Steroids, other Appearance and Performance Enhancing Drugs (APEDs), and other drugs of use and misuse, visit the NIDA website at www.drugabuse.gov or contact DrugPubs at 877-NIDA-NIH (877-643-2644; TTY/TDD: 240-645-0228).

NIDA's website includes:

- Information on drugs of use and misuse and related health consequences

- NIDA publications, news, and events

- Resources for health care professionals, educators, and patients and families

- Information on NIDA research studies and clinical trials

- Funding information (including program announcements and deadlines)

- International activities

- Links to related websites (access to websites of many other organizations in the field)

- Information in Spanish (en español)

NIDA websites and webpages

- drugabuse.gov/publications/drugfacts/anabolic-steroids

- drugabuse.gov/drugs-abuse/steroids-anabolic

- drugabuse.gov

- teens.drugabuse.gov

- easyread.drugabuse.gov

- researchstudies.drugabuse.gov

- irp.drugabuse.gov

For physician information

- NIDAMED: drugabuse.gov/nidamed

Other websites

Information on the abuse of Steroids and other Appearance and Performance Enhancing Drugs (APEDs) is also available through the following websites:

- Monitoring the Future

- The Partnership for Drug-Free Kids

- World Anti-Doping Agency:

- Labeling information from the FDA: Testosterone labeling

- Labeling information from the FDA: Tainted Products Marketed as Dietary Supplements

- Steroid prevention programs for high school athletes: Athletes Training & Learning to Avoid Steroids (ATLAS)

- Steroid prevention programs for high school athletes: Athletes Targeting Healthy Exercise & Nutrition Alternatives (ATHENA)

References

1. Kanayama G, Pope HG. History and epidemiology of anabolic androgens in athletes and non-athletes. *Mol Cell Endocrinol*. March 2017. doi:10.1016/j.mce.2017.02.039

2. Rashid H, Ormerod S, Day E. Anabolic androgenic steroids: what the psychiatrist needs to know. *Adv Psychiatr Treat*. 2007;13(3):203-211.

3. Lipsett MB, Korenman SG. Androgen Metabolism. *JAMA*. 1964;190(8):757-762. doi:10.1001/jama.1964.03070210063011

4. Shahidi NT. A review of the chemistry, biological action, and clinical applications of anabolic-androgenic steroids. *Clin Ther*. 2001;23(9):1355-1390.

5. FDA. Testosterone Information. https://www.fda.gov/drugs/drugsafety/postmarketdrugsafetyinformationforp Published March 3, 2015. Accessed May 26, 2017.

6. Rao PK, Boulet SL, Mehta A, et al. Trends in Testosterone Replacement Therapy Use from 2003 to 2013 among Reproductive-Age Men in the United States. *J Urol*. 2017;197(4):1121-1126. doi:10.1016/j.juro.2016.10.063.

7. Brennan R, Wells JSG, Van Hout MC. The injecting use of image and performance-enhancing drugs (IPED) in the general population: a systematic review. *Health Soc Care Community*. January 2016. doi:10.1111/hsc.12326.

8. Hildebrandt T, Langenbucher JW, Carr SJ, Sanjuan P. Modeling population heterogeneity in appearance- and performance-enhancing drug (APED) use: applications of mixture modeling in 400 regular APED users. *J Abnorm Psychol*. 2007;116(4):717-733. doi:10.1037/0021-843X.116.4.71.

9. Gennaro MC, Abrigo C. Caffeine and theobromine in coffee, tea and cola-beverages. *Fresenius J Anal Chem*. 1992;343(6):523-525.

10. NCCIH. Ephedra. NCCIH. https://nccih.nih.gov/health/ephedra. Published November 9, 2011. Accessed November 6, 2017.

11. Office of Dietary Supplements.
    Ephedra. https://ods.od.nih.gov/Health_Information/Ephedra.aspx.
    Published n.d. Accessed December 13, 2017.

12. American Thyroid Association. Thyroid and Weight FAQ. June
    2012. http://www.thyroid.org/thyroid-and-weight/. Accessed November 6,
    2017.

13. 108th Congress FS. *Regulation of Dietary Supplements: Hearing Before the
    Committee on Commerce, Science and Transportation.*;
    2003. https://www.gpo.gov/fdsys/pkg/CHRG-108shrg20196/pdf/CHRG-
    108shrg20196.pdf. Accessed February 7, 2018.

14. 108th Congress. *Anabolic Steroid Control Act of 2004.* Vol S.2195.;
    2004. https://www.congress.gov/bill/108th-congress/senate-bill/2195/all-
    info. Accessed April 28, 2017.

15. Freeman ER, Bloom DA, McGuire EJ. A brief history of testosterone. *J Urol.*
    2001;165(2):371-373. doi:10.1097/00005392-200102000-00004.

16. Altschule MD, Tillotson KJ. The use of testosterone in the treatment of
    depressions. *N Engl J Med.* 1948;239(27):1036-1038.
    doi:10.1056/NEJM194812302392704.

17. Wade N. Anabolic Steroids: Doctors Denounce Them, but Athletes Aren't
    Listening. *Science.* 1972;176(4042):1399-1403.
    doi:10.1126/science.176.4042.1399.

18. Buckley WE, Yesalis CE, Friedl KE, Anderson WA, Streit AL, Wright JE.
    Estimated prevalence of anabolic steroid use among male high school
    seniors. *JAMA.* 1988;260(23):3441-3445.

19. Pope HG, Kouri EM, Hudson JI. Effects of supraphysiologic doses of
    testosterone on mood and aggression in normal men: a randomized
    controlled trial. *Arch Gen Psychiatry.* 2000;57(2):133-140; discussion 155-
    156.

20. FDA. Significant Dates in U.S. Food and Drug Law History.
    2014. http://www.fda.gov/aboutfda/whatwedo/history/milestones/ucm128305.htm.
    Accessed June 4, 2016.

21. DEA. A Dangerous and Illegal Way to Seek Athletic Dominance and Better

Appearance - A Guide for Understanding the Dangers of Anabolic Steroids. March 2004. https://www.deadiversion.usdoj.gov/pubs/brochures/steroids/public/. Accessed April 25, 2017.

22. Kanayama G, Boynes M, Hudson JI, Field AE, Pope HG. Anabolic steroid abuse among teenage girls: an illusory problem? *Drug Alcohol Depend.* 2007;88(2-3):156-162. doi:10.1016/j.drugalcdep.2006.10.013.

23. Pope HG, Kanayama G, Athey A, Ryan E, Hudson JI, Baggish A. The lifetime prevalence of anabolic-androgenic steroid use and dependence in Americans: current best estimates. *Am J Addict Am Acad Psychiatr Alcohol Addict.* 2014;23(4):371-377. doi:10.1111/j.1521-0391.2013.12118.x.

24. Irving LM, Wall M, Neumark-Sztainer D, Story M. Steroid use among adolescents: findings from Project EAT. *J Adolesc Health Off Publ Soc Adolesc Med.* 2002;30(4):243-252.

25. Pope HG, Khalsa JH, Bhasin S. Body Image Disorders and Abuse of Anabolic-Androgenic Steroids Among Men. *JAMA.* 2017;317(1):23-24. doi:10.1001/jama.2016.17441.

26. Ip EJ, Barnett MJ, Tenerowicz MJ, Perry PJ. The Anabolic 500 survey: characteristics of male users versus nonusers of anabolic-androgenic steroids for strength training. *Pharmacotherapy.* 2011;31(8):757-766. doi:10.1592/phco.31.8.757.

27. Gruber AJ, Pope HG. Compulsive weight lifting and anabolic drug abuse among women rape victims. *Compr Psychiatry.* 1999;40(4):273-277.

28. Wright S, Grogan S, Hunter G. Motivations for Anabolic Steroid use Among Bodybuilders. *J Health Psychol.* 2000;5(4):566-571. doi:10.1177/135910530000500413.

29. American Academy of Pediatrics. Adolescents and anabolic steroids: a subject review. American Academy of Pediatrics. Committee on Sports Medicine and Fitness. *Pediatrics.* 1997;99(6):904-908.

30. Bahrke MS, Wright JE, Strauss RH, Catlin DH. Psychological moods and subjectively perceived behavioral and somatic changes accompanying anabolic-androgenic steroid use. *Am J Sports Med.* 1992;20(6):717-724.

31. Beiner JM, Jokl P, Cholewicki J, Panjabi MM. The effect of anabolic steroids and corticosteroids on healing of muscle contusion injury. *Am J Sports Med.* 1999;27(1):2-9.

32. Ferry A, Noirez P, Page CL, Salah IB, Daegelen D, Rieu M. Effects of anabolic/androgenic steroids on regenerating skeletal muscles in the rat. *Acta Physiol Scand.* 1999;166(2):105-110. doi:10.1046/j.1365-201x.1999.00549.x.

33. Ferry A, Vignaud A, Noirez P, Bertucci W. Respective effects of anabolic/androgenic steroids and physical exercise on isometric contractile properties of regenerating skeletal muscles in the rat. *Arch Physiol Biochem.* 2000;108(3):257-261. doi:10.1076/1381345520000710831ZFT257.

34. Eklöf A-C, Thurelius A-M, Garle M, Rane A, Sjöqvist F. The anti-doping hot-line, a means to capture the abuse of doping agents in the Swedish society and a new service function in clinical pharmacology. *Eur J Clin Pharmacol.* 2003;59(8-9):571-577. doi:10.1007/s00228-003-0633-z.

35. Medline Plus. Testosterone Topical. June 2016. https://www.nlm.nih.gov/medlineplus/druginfo/meds/a605020.html#why.

36. Trenton AJ, Currier GW. Behavioural manifestations of anabolic steroid use. *CNS Drugs.* 2005;19(7):571-595.

37. Evans NA. Gym and tonic: a profile of 100 male steroid users. *Br J Sports Med.* 1997;31(1):54-58.

38. Wilson JD. Androgen abuse by athletes. *Endocr Rev.* 1988;9(2):181-199. doi:10.1210/edrv-9-2-181.

39. Frati P, Busardò FP, Cipolloni L, Dominicis ED, Fineschi V. Anabolic Androgenic Steroid (AAS) related deaths: autoptic, histopathological and toxicological findings. *Curr Neuropharmacol.* 2015;13(1):146-159. doi:10.2174/1570159X13666141210225414.

40. Bronson FH, Matherne CM. Exposure to anabolic-androgenic steroids shortens life span of male mice. *Med Sci Sports Exerc.* 1997;29(5):615-619.

41. Urhausen A, Albers T, Kindermann W. Are the cardiac effects of anabolic steroid abuse in strength athletes reversible? *Heart Br Card Soc.* 2004;90(5):496-501.

42. Kaskutas LA. Alcoholics anonymous effectiveness: faith meets science. *J Addict Dis*. 2009;28(2):145-157. doi:10.1080/10550880902772464.

43. Vanberg P, Atar D. Androgenic anabolic steroid abuse and the cardiovascular system. *Handb Exp Pharmacol*. 2010;(195):411-457. doi:10.1007/978-3-540-79088-4_18.

44. Baggish AL, Weiner RB, Kanayama G, et al. Cardiovascular Toxicity of Illicit Anabolic-Androgenic Steroid Use. *Circulation*. 2017;135(21):1991-2002. doi:10.1161/CIRCULATIONAHA.116.026945.

45. El Scheich T, Weber A-A, Klee D, Schweiger D, Mayatepek E, Karenfort M. Adolescent ischemic stroke associated with anabolic steroid and cannabis abuse. *J Pediatr Endocrinol Metab JPEM*. 2013;26(1-2):161-165. doi:10.1515/jpem-2012-0057.

46. Santamarina RD, Besocke AG, Romano LM, Ioli PL, Gonorazky SE. Ischemic stroke related to anabolic abuse. *Clin Neuropharmacol*. 2008;31(2):80-85. doi:10.1097/WNF.0b013e3180ed4485.

47. Palatini P, Giada F, Garavelli G, et al. Cardiovascular effects of anabolic steroids in weight-trained subjects. *J Clin Pharmacol*. 1996;36(12):1132-1140.

48. Bhasin S, Woodhouse L, Casaburi R, et al. Testosterone dose-response relationships in healthy young men. *Am J Physiol Endocrinol Metab*. 2001;281(6):E1172-1181.

49. Linton MF, Yancey PG, Davies SS, Jerome WG (Jay), Linton EF, Vickers KC. The Role of Lipids and Lipoproteins in Atherosclerosis. In: De Groot LJ, Chrousos G, Dungan K, et al., eds. *Endotext*. South Dartmouth (MA): MDText.com, Inc.; 2000. http://www.ncbi.nlm.nih.gov/books/NBK343489/. Accessed April 21, 2017.

50. Robles-Diaz M, Gonzalez-Jimenez A, Medina-Caliz I, et al. Distinct phenotype of hepatotoxicity associated with illicit use of anabolic androgenic steroids. *Aliment Pharmacol Ther*. 2015;41(1):116-125. doi:10.1111/apt.13023.

51. Schwingel PA, Cotrim HP, Santos CR dos, et al. Recreational Anabolic-Androgenic Steroid Use Associated With Liver Injuries Among Brazilian Young Men. *Subst Use Misuse*. 2015;50(11):1490-1498.

doi:10.3109/10826084.2015.1018550.

52. Kosaka A, Takahashi H, Yajima Y, et al. Hepatocellular carcinoma associated with anabolic steroid therapy: report of a case and review of the Japanese literature. *J Gastroenterol*. 1996;31(3):450-454.

53. Socas L, Zumbado M, Pérez-Luzardo O, et al. Hepatocellular adenomas associated with anabolic androgenic steroid abuse in bodybuilders: a report of two cases and a review of the literature. *Br J Sports Med*. 2005;39(5):e27. doi:10.1136/bjsm.2004.013599.

54. Wakabayashi T, Onda H, Tada T, Iijima M, Itoh Y. High incidence of peliosis hepatis in autopsy cases of aplastic anemia with special reference to anabolic steroid therapy. *Acta Pathol Jpn*. 1984;34(5):1079-1086.

55. Hansma P, Diaz FJ, Njiwaji C. Fatal Liver Cyst Rupture Due to Anabolic Steroid Use: A Case Presentation. *Am J Forensic Med Pathol*. 2016;37(1):21-22. doi:10.1097/PAF.0000000000000218.

56. Bonetti A, Tirelli F, Catapano A, et al. Side effects of anabolic androgenic steroids abuse. *Int J Sports Med*. 2008;29(8):679-687. doi:10.1055/s-2007-965808.

57. Liu PY, Swerdloff RS, Christenson PD, Handelsman DJ, Wang C, Hormonal Male Contraception Summit Group. Rate, extent, and modifiers of spermatogenic recovery after hormonal male contraception: an integrated analysis. *Lancet Lond Engl*. 2006;367(9520):1412-1420. doi:10.1016/S0140-6736(06)68614-5.

58. Torres-Calleja J, González-Unzaga M, DeCelis-Carrillo R, Calzada-Sánchez L, Pedrón N. Effect of androgenic anabolic steroids on sperm quality and serum hormone levels in adult male bodybuilders. *Life Sci*. 2001;68(15):1769-1774.

59. Calzada L, Torres-Calleja J, Martinez JM, Pedrón N. Measurement of androgen and estrogen receptors in breast tissue from subjects with anabolic steroid-dependent gynecomastia. *Life Sci*. 2001;69(13):1465-1469.

60. Christou MA, Christou PA, Markozannes G, Tsatsoulis A, Mastorakos G, Tigas S. Effects of Anabolic Androgenic Steroids on the Reproductive System of Athletes and Recreational Users: A Systematic Review and Meta-

Analysis. *Sports Med Auckl NZ.* March 2017. doi:10.1007/s40279-017-0709-z.

61. Schürmeyer T, Knuth UA, Belkien L, Nieschlag E. Reversible azoospermia induced by the anabolic steroid 19-nortestosterone. *Lancet Lond Engl.* 1984;1(8374):417-420.

62. Orlandi MA, Venegoni E, Pagani C. Gynecomastia in two young men with histories of prolonged use of anabolic androgenic steroids. *J Ultrasound.* 2010;13(2):46-48. doi:10.1016/j.jus.2010.07.006.

63. Chimento A, Sirianni R, Zolea F, et al. Nandrolone and stanozolol induce Leydig cell tumor proliferation through an estrogen-dependent mechanism involving IGF-I system. *J Cell Physiol.* 2012;227(5):2079-2088. doi:10.1002/jcp.22936.

64. Baker J. A report on alterations to the speaking and singing voices of four women following hormonal therapy with virilizing agents. *J Voice Off J Voice Found.* 1999;13(4):496-507.

65. Scott MJ, Scott AM. Effects of anabolic-androgenic steroids on the pilosebaceous unit. *Cutis.* 1992;50(2):113-116.

66. Nieschlag E, Vorona E. MECHANISMS IN ENDOCRINOLOGY: Medical consequences of doping with anabolic androgenic steroids: effects on reproductive functions. *Eur J Endocrinol Eur Fed Endocr Soc.* 2015;173(2):R47-58. doi:10.1530/EJE-15-0080.

67. Zemel BS, Katz SH. The contribution of adrenal and gonadal androgens to the growth in height of adolescent males. *Am J Phys Anthropol.* 1986;71(4):459-466. doi:10.1002/ajpa.1330710409.

68. Bierich JR. Effects and side effects of anabolic steroids in children. *Acta Endocrinol Suppl (Copenh).* 1961;39(Suppl 63):89-110.

69. Seynnes OR, Kamandulis S, Kairaitis R, et al. Effect of androgenic-anabolic steroids and heavy strength training on patellar tendon morphological and mechanical properties. *J Appl Physiol Bethesda Md 1985.* 2013;115(1):84-89. doi:10.1152/japplphysiol.01417.2012.

70. Kraus SL, Emmert S, Schön MP, Haenssle HA. The dark side of beauty: acne fulminans induced by anabolic steroids in a male bodybuilder. *Arch*

Dermatol. 2012;148(10):1210-1212. doi:10.1001/archdermatol.2012.855.

71. Melnik B, Jansen T, Grabbe S. Abuse of anabolic-androgenic steroids and bodybuilding acne: an underestimated health problem. *J Dtsch Dermatol Ges J Ger Soc Dermatol JDDG.* 2007;5(2):110-117. doi:10.1111/j.1610-0387.2007.06176.x.

72. Voelcker V, Sticherling M, Bauerschmitz J. Severe ulcerated "bodybuilding acne" caused by anabolic steroid use and exacerbated by isotretinoin. *Int Wound J.* 2010;7(3):199-201. doi:10.1111/j.1742-481X.2010.00676.x.

73. Rich JD, Dickinson BP, Flanigan TP, Valone SE. Abscess related to anabolic-androgenic steroid injection. *Med Sci Sports Exerc.* 1999;31(2):207-209.

74. Cabb E, Baltar S, Powers DW, Mohan K, Martinez A, Pitts E. The Diagnosis and Manifestations of Liver Injury Secondary to Off-Label Androgenic Anabolic Steroid Use. *Case Rep Gastroenterol.* 2016;10(2):499-505. doi:10.1159/000448883.

75. Yoshida EM, Erb SR, Scudamore CH, Owen DA. Severe cholestasis and jaundice secondary to an esterified testosterone, a non-C17 alkylated anabolic steroid. *J Clin Gastroenterol.* 1994;18(3):268-270.

76. Ip EJ, Yadao MA, Shah BM, Lau B. Infectious disease, injection practices, and risky sexual behavior among anabolic steroid users. *AIDS Care.* 2016;28(3):294-299. doi:10.1080/09540121.2015.1090539.

77. Hughes TK, Fulep E, Juelich T, Smith EM, Stanton GJ. Modulation of immune responses by anabolic androgenic steroids. *Int J Immunopharmacol.* 1995;17(11):857-863.

78. Perry PJ, Kutscher EC, Lund BC, Yates WR, Holman TL, Demers L. Measures of aggression and mood changes in male weightlifters with and without androgenic anabolic steroid use. *J Forensic Sci.* 2003;48(3):646-651.

79. Lundholm L, Frisell T, Lichtenstein P, Långström N. Anabolic androgenic steroids and violent offending: confounding by polysubstance abuse among 10,365 general population men. *Addict Abingdon Engl.* 2015;110(1):100-108. doi:10.1111/add.12715.

80. Burnett KF, Kleiman ME. Psychological characteristics of adolescent steroid users. *Adolescence*. 1994;29(113):81-89.

81. Choi PY, Pope HG. Violence toward women and illicit androgenic-anabolic steroid use. *Ann Clin Psychiatry Off J Am Acad Clin Psychiatr*. 1994;6(1):21-25.

82. Daly RC, Su T-P, Schmidt PJ, Pagliaro M, Pickar D, Rubinow DR. Neuroendocrine and behavioral effects of high-dose anabolic steroid administration in male normal volunteers. *Psychoneuroendocrinology*. 2003;28(3):317-331.

83. Kouri EM, Lukas SE, Pope HG, Oliva PS. Increased aggressive responding in male volunteers following the administration of gradually increasing doses of testosterone cypionate. *Drug Alcohol Depend*. 1995;40(1):73-79.

84. Bahrke MS, Yesalis CE, Wright JE. Psychological and behavioural effects of endogenous testosterone and anabolic-androgenic steroids. An update. *Sports Med Auckl NZ*. 1996;22(6):367-390.

85. Tricker R, Casaburi R, Storer TW, et al. The effects of supraphysiological doses of testosterone on angry behavior in healthy eugonadal men--a clinical research center study. *J Clin Endocrinol Metab*. 1996;81(10):3754-3758. doi:10.1210/jcem.81.10.8855834.

86. Ip EJ, Lu DH, Barnett MJ, Tenerowicz MJ, Vo JC, Perry PJ. Psychological and physical impact of anabolic-androgenic steroid dependence. *Pharmacotherapy*. 2012;32(10):910-919. doi:10.1002/j.1875-9114.2012.01123.

87. Pope HG, Katz DL. Psychiatric and medical effects of anabolic-androgenic steroid use. A controlled study of 160 athletes. *Arch Gen Psychiatry*. 1994;51(5):375-382.

88. Kanayama G, Pope HG. Illicit use of androgens and other hormones: recent advances. *Curr Opin Endocrinol Diabetes Obes*. 2012;19(3):211-219. doi:10.1097/MED.0b013e3283524008.

89. Kanayama G, Cohane GH, Weiss RD, Pope HG. Past anabolic-androgenic steroid use among men admitted for substance abuse treatment: an underrecognized problem? *J Clin Psychiatry*. 2003;64(2):156-160.

90. Wines JD, Gruber AJ, Pope HG, Lukas SE. Nalbuphine hydrochloride dependence in anabolic steroid users. *Am J Addict.* 1999;8(2):161-164.

91. Arvary D, Pope HG. Anabolic-androgenic steroids as a gateway to opioid dependence. *N Engl J Med.* 2000;342(20):1532. doi:10.1056/NEJM200005183422018.

92. Keenan BS, Richards GE, Ponder SW, Dallas JS, Nagamani M, Smith ER. Androgen-stimulated pubertal growth: the effects of testosterone and dihydrotestosterone on growth hormone and insulin-like growth factor-I in the treatment of short stature and delayed puberty. *J Clin Endocrinol Metab.* 1993;76(4):996-1001. doi:10.1210/jcem.76.4.8473416.

93. Morris JA, Jordan CL, Breedlove SM. Sexual differentiation of the vertebrate nervous system. *Nat Neurosci.* 2004;7(10):1034-1039. doi:10.1038/nn1325.

94. Romeo RD, Richardson HN, Sisk CL. Puberty and the maturation of the male brain and sexual behavior: recasting a behavioral potential. *Neurosci Biobehav Rev.* 2002;26(3):381-391.

95. Schulz KM, Molenda-Figueira HA, Sisk CL. Back to the future: The organizational-activational hypothesis adapted to puberty and adolescence. *Horm Behav.* 2009;55(5):597-604. doi:10.1016/j.yhbeh.2009.03.010.

96. Zehr JL, Nichols LR, Schulz KM, Sisk CL. Adolescent development of neuron structure in dentate gyrus granule cells of male Syrian hamsters. *Dev Neurobiol.* 2008;68(14):1517-1526. doi:10.1002/dneu.20675.

97. Cunningham RL, Claiborne BJ, McGinnis MY. Pubertal exposure to anabolic androgenic steroids increases spine densities on neurons in the limbic system of male rats. *Neuroscience.* 2007;150(3):609-615. doi:10.1016/j.neuroscience.2007.09.038.

98. Hildebrandt T, Langenbucher JW, Flores A, Harty S, Berlin HA, Berlin H. The influence of age of onset and acute anabolic steroid exposure on cognitive performance, impulsivity, and aggression in men. *Psychol Addict Behav J Soc Psychol Addict Behav.* 2014;28(4):1096-1104. doi:10.1037/a0036482.

99. Olivares EL, Silveira ALB, Fonseca FV, et al. Administration of an anabolic steroid during the adolescent phase changes the behavior, cardiac

autonomic balance and fluid intake in male adult rats. *Physiol Behav.* 2014;126:15-24. doi:10.1016/j.physbeh.2013.12.006.

100. Grimes JM, Melloni RH. Prolonged alterations in the serotonin neural system following the cessation of adolescent anabolic-androgenic steroid exposure in hamsters (Mesocricetus auratus). *Behav Neurosci.* 2006;120(6):1242-1251. doi:10.1037/0735-7044.120.6.1242.

101. Ricci LA, Rasakham K, Grimes JM, Melloni RH. Serotonin-1A receptor activity and expression modulate adolescent anabolic/androgenic steroid-induced aggression in hamsters. *Pharmacol Biochem Behav.* 2006;85(1):1-11. doi:10.1016/j.pbb.2006.06.022.

102. Menard CS, Harlan RE. Up-regulation of androgen receptor immunoreactivity in the rat brain by androgenic-anabolic steroids. *Brain Res.* 1993;622(1-2):226-236.

103. Matsumoto T, Sakari M, Okada M, et al. The androgen receptor in health and disease. *Annu Rev Physiol.* 2013;75:201-224. doi:10.1146/annurev-physiol-030212-183656.

104. Vicencio JM, Estrada M, Galvis D, et al. Anabolic androgenic steroids and intracellular calcium signaling: a mini review on mechanisms and physiological implications. *Mini Rev Med Chem.* 2011;11(5):390-398.

105. Yang P, Jones BL, Henderson LP. Mechanisms of anabolic androgenic steroid modulation of alpha(1)beta(3)gamma(2L) GABA(A) receptors. *Neuropharmacology.* 2002;43(4):619-633.

106. Yang P, Jones BL, Henderson LP. Role of the alpha subunit in the modulation of GABA(A) receptors by anabolic androgenic steroids. *Neuropharmacology.* 2005;49(3):300-316. doi:10.1016/j.neuropharm.2005.03.017.

107. Kindlundh AM, Lindblom J, Bergström L, Wikberg JE, Nyberg F. The anabolic-androgenic steroid nandrolone decanoate affects the density of dopamine receptors in the male rat brain. *Eur J Neurosci.* 2001;13(2):291-296.

108. Thiblin I, Finn A, Ross SB, Stenfors C. Increased dopaminergic and 5-hydroxytryptaminergic activities in male rat brain following long-term treatment with anabolic androgenic steroids. *Br J Pharmacol.*

1999;126(6):1301-1306. doi:10.1038/sj.bjp.0702412.

109. Zotti M, Tucci P, Colaianna M, et al. Chronic nandrolone administration induces dysfunction of the reward pathway in rats. *Steroids*. 2014;79:7-13.

110. Kanayama G, Brower KJ, Wood RI, Hudson JI, Pope HG. Issues for DSM-V: clarifying the diagnostic criteria for anabolic-androgenic steroid dependence. *Am J Psychiatry*. 2009;166(6):642-645. doi:10.1176/appi.ajp.2009.08111699.

111. Brower KJ, Blow FC, Young JP, Hill EM. Symptoms and correlates of anabolic-androgenic steroid dependence. *Br J Addict*. 1991;86(6):759-768.

112. Malone DA, Dimeff RJ, Lombardo JA, Sample RH. Psychiatric effects and psychoactive substance use in anabolic-androgenic steroid users. *Clin J Sport Med Off J Can Acad Sport Med*. 1995;5(1):25-31.

113. WADA. *2015 Anti-Doping Rule Violations (ADRVs) Report.*; 2017. https://www.wada-ama.org/sites/default/files/resources/files/2015_adrvs_report_web_release_0.pdf.

114. WADA. Compliance Monitoring. https://www.wada-ama.org/en/questions-answers/compliance-monitoring. Published 2017. Accessed May 18, 2017.

115. Geyer H, Schänzer W, Thevis M. Anabolic agents: recent strategies for their detection and protection from inadvertent doping. *Br J Sports Med*. 2014;48(10):820-826. doi:10.1136/bjsports-2014-093526.

116. Catlin DH, Sekera MH, Ahrens BD, Starcevic B, Chang Y-C, Hatton CK. Tetrahydrogestrinone: discovery, synthesis, and detection in urine. *Rapid Commun Mass Spectrom RCM*. 2004;18(12):1245-1049. doi:10.1002/rcm.1495.

117. Catlin DH, Ahrens BD, Kucherova Y. Detection of norbolethone, an anabolic steroid never marketed, in athletes' urine. *Rapid Commun Mass Spectrom RCM*. 2002;16(13):1273-1275. doi:10.1002/rcm.722.

118. Sekera MH, Ahrens BD, Chang Y-C, Starcevic B, Georgakopoulos C, Catlin DH. Another designer steroid: discovery, synthesis, and detection of "madol" in urine. *Rapid Commun Mass Spectrom RCM*. 2005;19(6):781-784. doi:10.1002/rcm.1858.

119. Mareck U, Geyer H, Opfermann G, Thevis M, Schänzer W. Factors

influencing the steroid profile in doping control analysis. *J Mass Spectrom JMS*. 2008;43(7):877-891. doi:10.1002/jms.1457.

120. Yonamine M, Garcia PR, de Moraes Moreau RL. Non-intentional doping in sports. *Sports Med Auckl NZ*. 2004;34(11):697-704.

121. Jung J, Hermanns-Clausen M, Weinmann W. Anorectic sibutramine detected in a Chinese herbal drug for weight loss. *Forensic Sci Int*. 2006;161(2-3):221-222. doi:10.1016/j.forsciint.2006.02.052.

122. Parr MK, Koehler K, Geyer H, Guddat S, Schänzer W. Clenbuterol marketed as dietary supplement. *Biomed Chromatogr BMC*. 2008;22(3):298-300. doi:10.1002/bmc.928.

123. Geyer H, Braun H, Burke LM, Stear SJ, Castell LM. A-Z of nutritional supplements: dietary supplements, sports nutrition foods and ergogenic aids for health and performance--Part 22. *Br J Sports Med*. 2011;45(9):752-754. doi:10.1136/bjsports-2011-090180.

124. De Cock KJ, Delbeke FT, Van Eenoo P, Desmet N, Roels K, De Backer P. Detection and determination of anabolic steroids in nutritional supplements. *J Pharm Biomed Anal*. 2001;25(5-6):843-852.

125. FDA. Tainted Products Marketed as Dietary Supplements. https://www.accessdata.fda.gov/scripts/sda/sdNavigation.cfm?sd=tainted_supplements_cder. Accessed January 9, 2018.

126. WADA. World Anti-Doping Code. 2009. https://www.wada-ama.org/sites/default/files/resources/files/wada_anti-doping_code_2009_en_0.pdf. Accessed May 23, 2017.

127. Elliot D, Goldberg L. Intervention and prevention of steroid use in adolescents. *Am J Sports Med*. 1996;24(6 Suppl):S46-47.

128. Goldberg L, Bents R, Bosworth E, Trevisan L, Elliot DL. Anabolic steroid education and adolescents: do scare tactics work? *Pediatrics*. 1991;87(3):283-286.

129. Middleman AB, Faulkner AH, Woods ER, Emans SJ, DuRant RH. High-risk behaviors among high school students in Massachusetts who use anabolic steroids. *Pediatrics*. 1995;96(2 Pt 1):268-272.

130. Goldberg L, MacKinnon DP, Elliot DL, Moe EL, Clarke G, Cheong J. The

adolescents training and learning to avoid steroids program: preventing drug use and promoting health behaviors. *Arch Pediatr Adolesc Med.* 2000;154(4):332-338.

131. Elliot DL, Goldberg L, Moe EL, Defrancesco CA, Durham MB, Hix-Small H. Preventing substance use and disordered eating: initial outcomes of the ATHENA (athletes targeting healthy exercise and nutrition alternatives) program. *Arch Pediatr Adolesc Med.* 2004;158(11):1043-1049. doi:10.1001/archpedi.158.11.1043.

132. Elliot DL, Goldberg L, Moe EL, et al. Long-term Outcomes of the ATHENA (Athletes Targeting Healthy Exercise & Nutrition Alternatives) Program for Female High School Athletes. *J Alcohol Drug Educ.* 2008;52(2):73-92.

133. Pope HG, Kanayama G, Ionescu-Pioggia M, Hudson JI. Anabolic steroid users' attitudes towards physicians. *Addict Abingdon Engl.* 2004;99(9):1189-1194. doi:10.1111/j.1360-0443.2004.00781.x.

134. Brennan BP, Kanayama G, Pope HG. Performance-enhancing drugs on the web: a growing public-health issue. *Am J Addict Am Acad Psychiatr Alcohol Addict.* 2013;22(2):158-161. doi:10.1111/j.1521-0391.2013.00311.x.

135. Kanayama G, Brower KJ, Wood RI, Hudson JI, Pope HG. Treatment of anabolic-androgenic steroid dependence: Emerging evidence and its implications. *Drug Alcohol Depend.* 2010;109(1-3):6-13. doi:10.1016/j.drugalcdep.2010.01.011